INTERMITTENT FASTING

Burn Fat, Lose Weight And Build Muscle With Ease While Still Eating Your Favorite Foods!

Gerard Hamilton

Medical Disclaimer: This book does not contain any medical advice. The ideas and suggestions contained in this book are not intended as a substitute for consulting with your doctor. All matters regarding your health require medical supervision.

Legal Disclaimer: all photos used in this book are licensed for commercial use or in the public domain.

ERRORS

Please contact me if you find any errors.

My publisher and I have taken every effort to ensure the quality and correctness of this book. However, after going over the book draft time and again, we sometimes don't see the forest for the trees anymore.

If you notice any errors, I would really appreciate it if you could contact me directly before taking any other action. This allows me to quickly fix it.

Errors: errors@semsoli.com

REVIEWS

Reviews and feedback help improve this book and the author.

If you enjoy this book, I would greatly appreciate it if you were able to take a few moments to share your opinion and post a review online.

By the Same Author

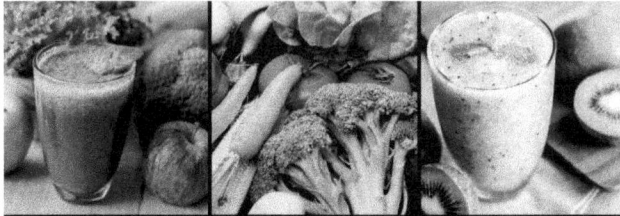

JUICING
FOR BEGINNERS

FEEL GREAT AGAIN WITH THESE
50 WEIGHT LOSS RECIPES

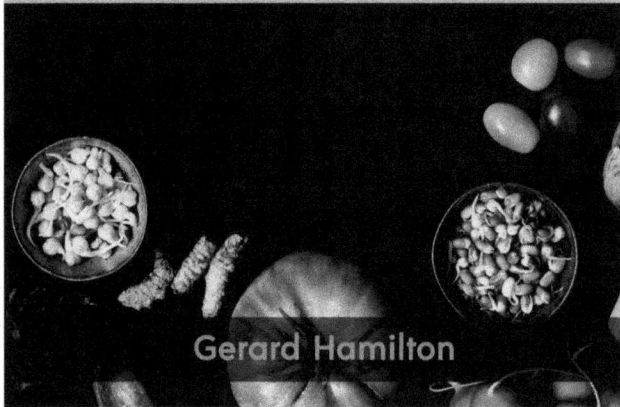

Gerard Hamilton

Table of Contents

Introduction..10

1. What is Intermittent Fasting............................14
      Intermittent Fasting 101
      Fasting Throughout the Ages
      Different Techniques Depending On Needs
      When To Eat And Not What To Eat
      You Can Consume Beverages, With No Calories

2. Health Benefits Of Intermittent Fasting............20
      Helps Losing Weight And Belly Fat
      Reduces Risk of Cancer
      Positive Changes In Cell Functioning
      Reduces Insulin Resistance
      Reduces Stress and Inflammation
      It's Good For Your Heart
      Slows Down Aging

3. Intermittent Fasting Methods: Which One Is Right For You?..26
      16:8 Method (Leangains)
      5:2 Method
      Eat-Stop-Eat
      Alternate Day Fasting
      Warrior Diet
      Skipping Meals Spontaneously

4. Who Should Not Fast?........................34
    Eating Disorders
    Pregnant Women
    Type 2 Diabetes
    Other Medical Conditions
    Before and After Surgery
    Mental Fear of Fasting
    Children

5. Common Fasting Myths Debunked....................40
    Myth#1: You Will Become Fat If You Skip Breakfast
    Myth#2: Eating Frequently Will Boost Your Metabolism
    Myth#3: Hunger Reduces If You Eat Frequently
    Myth#4: Small Meals Can Help You Lose Weight
    Myth#5: Your Brain Requires A Constant Supply Of Glucose
    Myth#6: Your Body Will Shift To Starvation Mode
    Myth#7: Your Body Can Only Make Use Of A Limited Amount Of Consumed Protein
    Myth#8: You Will Lose Muscle
    Myth#9: It's Bad For Your Health
    Myth#10: When You Are Not Fasting, You Will Overeat

6. What Can You Consume During the Fasting Window..50
    Water/Tea
    Coffee
    Avoid Insulin Spikes
    No Chewing Gum

No Diet drinks

No Alcohol

7. How To Get Started – 10 Steps To Create Your Intermittent Fasting Plan..56

Step 1: Select The Method Of Fasting

Step 2: Do Plenty Of Research

Step 3: Get The Tools

Step 4: Start The Transition

Step 5: Find The Necessary Support

Step 6: Tone Down Your Workouts

Step 7: Follow Delayed Gratification

Step 8: Protein Should Be A Priority

Step 9: Take A "Before" Photograph

Step 10: One More Thing To Keep In Mind

8. Intermittent Fasting Plan Templates..................66

Write Down Your Goals

16:8 Method (Leangains)

5:2 Method / Eat – Stop – Eat

The Warrior Diet Method

9. How To Stay On Track and Motivated.................72

Don't Expect Results Overnight

Use Positive Affirmations

Measure Your Progress Using a Mirror Instead of a Scale

Partner Up

Eat Healthy, Delicious Foods

Stay Calm and Keep it Cool

Do Not Worry About People Staring at You

Keep Yourself Busy
Always Listen To Your Body

Final Words..82

Resources..84
Books
Websites
Documentaries
Podcasts

BONUS CHAPTER: The Health Benefits of Juicing..86
Introduction
Juicing Slows Down Aging
Juicing Makes You Look Better
Juicing Helps You Lose Weight
Juicing Increases Your Energy Level
Juicing Boosts Your Immune System

Did You Like This Book?......................................94

About The Author..96

Introduction

Thank you for taking the time to purchase this book: *'Intermittent Fasting: Burn Fat, Lose Weight And Build Muscle With Ease While Still Eating Your Favorite Foods!'*

Welcome to this <u>2nd edition</u>, which has been completely revised and updated in <u>December 2018</u>.

When did you have your last meal? Was it an hour ago, or several hours ago? Was it yesterday? Do you feel like you are going to die out of starvation?

Most of us would have felt like that at one point in time or the other. Even after eating, we end up feeling a little hungry after a while. Well, intermittent fasting will help you in understanding your body and your hunger pangs. It will allow you to understand that hunger has got a peak point, and after that, it disappears. After a while, even though you haven't had anything to eat for hours, you will not feel hungry.

One thing you need to understand is that intermittent fasting is not a diet. It divides your time in two windows: one in which you are allowed to consume calories, and one in which you are not.

Intermittent fasting helps you in cutting down what you eat, but ensures that you have got your daily calorie requirement through wholesome meals.

Here is what it might look like:

- you skip breakfast every day;
- eat two healthy meals after spaced intervals at around 1 pm and 8 pm.

That's about it.

Does this make you cringe in horror? How can you just survive on two meals? How will your metabolism cope with this? Will your workout routine go for a toss?

Relax. You won't pass out by the end of the day!

Even though these days most people have a pattern of eating every couple of hours, human beings haven't always had this luxury. For most of our history, human beings had to find food first before they could eat it. They were fasting at intervals without even trying to, yet they survived. Our body's can easily adapt to not eating for certain periods of time. And as a matter of fact; you are already practicing intermittent fasting! Each time when you go to bed and then wake up in the morning, you don't eat anything for about 8 hours. By consciously practicing intermittent fasting, you are simply prolonging this window.

In this book, we will discuss the most important ways in which you can go about fasting. Simply pick the one that best fits your needs and lifestyle. Whichever one you choose; all will result in amazing health benefits!

Over a period of time, intermittent fasting will help to reduce your body fat, as well as get you back in shape. You will also be able to control your hunger pangs. If you were amongst those who are conscious about their fitness and eat three meals a day or manage about 5-6 small meals, then the thought of fasting would scare you. If you are an active person then you may get the urge to eat after every five or six hours.

Once you start reading this book, you will realize that you won't die of starvation or lose your muscle. You will just shed the excess body fat.

Intermittent fasting also helps in getting the body's insulin and glucose levels under control.

And one final thing that I can promise you is that you will be liberated from this fear of wasting away if you don't eat every few hours. Depending on the fasting plan that you are opting for, you will have to plan your meals. Intermittent fasting will help in getting your body under your control.

So: Are you ready to shake things up in your life? In a good way!

Now is the day on which you can take the **first step** to **taking back control** of your **health**.

Are you ready?

1. What is Intermittent Fasting

"I feel so much better on it. I haven't put on nearly the amount of fat I normally would. And the great thing about this diet is, I sleep so much better."

Hugh Jackman, of Wolverine fame, on how intermittent fasting helps him bulk and cut for movie roles.

*<u>**Key Takeaway**</u>: Intermittent Fasting is a form of dieting where one alternates between periods of absolute fasting and eating. This form of fasting has many health benefits. Also, it doesn't place any constraints on what you have to eat and what you don't.*

Intermittent fasting seems to be the recent fad that has taken over the world of fitness trends. Intermittent fasting involves oscillating between periods of fasting and eating. There are studies that show that this diet can indeed facilitate weight loss, improve immunity, and promote your metabolism as well. In this chapter, you will learn what intermittent fasting is all about.

***

Intermittent Fasting 101

Intermittent fasting is about alternating between periods of eating and fasting. The focus isn't so much on the kind of foods you should consume; instead, the focus is on when you should eat.

You might have never thought of it, but everyone fasts every day. When you are getting your ZZZs! Think of intermittent fasting as a simple extension of that fasting period.

There are different methods of intermittent fasting. The 16:8 method is perhaps the most common one. With this method, you are fasting for about 16 hours in a day. Your eating window is restricted to an 8-hour cycle. For example, you skip your breakfast; have your first meal at noon and the last one at 8pm. Later on in this book, we will discuss the most popular intermittent fasting methods.

Notwithstanding what people usually assume, intermittent fasting is relatively easy to follow. Hunger can be tackled easily. Initially it might be tough to get used to it, however, with the passage of time, it does get easier.

You aren't allowed to consume any food during the fasting period. A couple of beverages like coffee and tea are allowed though, in moderation. Some forms of intermittent fasting also provide for the consumption of low-calorie foods in small amounts during the fast period. Supplements can be consumed, provided they don't add any calories.

Fasting Throughout the Ages

The concept of fasting isn't a new one. Human beings have been doing this since forever, often out of necessity due to lack of food. Our bodies have been designed in such a way that they can go for long periods of time without any food.

Intermittent fasting is also prominent in all major religions, and is used as a way to humble one self and experience closer intimacy with God:

- **Christianity**: Jesus fasted for forty days and nights in preparation for his ministry.
- **Islam**: During Ramadan, Muslims fast from dawn until sunset for one month, to commemorate the revelation of the Quran to Muhammad.
- **Judaism**: The Fast of the Firstborn commemorates the salvation of the Israelite firstborns during the last of the ten plagues, when all Egyptian firstborns were killed. Usually this fast falls on the day before Passover. Interestingly enough, only firstborns are required to fast on this day.
- **Buddhism**: Buddhist monks and nuns practice intermittent fasting every day. They follow the Vinaya rules, a code of discipline laid down by the Buddha himself. One of the rules in this code is to not eat anything after the noon meal.

- **Hinduism**: Fasting is very prominent among Hindus. The type of fast, and when it is done, depends on personal belief, as well as which deity one favors.

***

Different Techniques Depending On Needs

There is not just one way of doing a fast. Intermittent fasting might mean different things for different people. In Chapter 3, we will discuss the most common fasting methods.

A little teaser: besides the 16:8 method we just talked about, another common one is the 5:2 method is. If you were following this approach, you would fast for two nonconsecutive days in the week. The rest of the days, there is no restriction on the number of calories that you can consume.

Ultimately, you will perform at your highest level on a fast that best fits your needs and lifestyle.

***

When To Eat And Not What To Eat

Intermittent fasting is not a diet: there is caloric constraint on those who follow it. The plans for this diet can be personalized quite easily. It focuses more on the *time at which* you can eat and not *what* you eat. What matters is that you adhere to the fasting window.

With that being said, it is always good to limit your processed foods intake. Not only is eating junk food not good for your health, it will also worsen your food cravings during the fasting window as you are not giving your body the nutrients it needs. Instead, aim to consume healthy focus on healthy fats (raw nuts, avocados, olive or coconut oil, salmon), proteins (meat, eggs, lentils) and leafy vegetables.

Don't get disheartened if this sounds a bit intense right now. Just try out one method for a while, and if it doesn't work for you, experiment with a different one. You will find one method that works best for you.

***

You Can Consume Beverages, With No Calories

There is one exception when it comes to fasting: you can drink water! All you have been told is to avoid consuming any food with calories in it. You may also drink other liquids like tea and black coffee, as long as it does not contain any calories. That means no cream or sugar!

***

These are the basics of intermittent fasting. Now let's take a look at the many health benefits that are associated with intermittent fasting.

2. Health Benefits Of Intermittent Fasting

"To insure good health: eat lightly, breathe deeply, live moderately, cultivate cheerfulness, and maintain an interest in life."

William Londen

Key Takeaway*: There are many health benefits to Intermittent Fasting and all of them are related to not consuming food for some time. Fasting allows for change in the functioning of your cells and helps in cell repair. Other than that, Intermittent Fasting also helps you to lose weight.*

Limiting your food consumption to a strict time window, while fasting for the remainder of the time, is associated with many health benefits.

Your body needs to burn energy to digest the food you eat. If you eat something every couple of hours, your body is continuously in food-digestion mode. However, if you practice intermittent fasting, your body can use that same energy for maintenance during the fasting window. Isn't it telling that animals and human beings alike tend to fast when they fall sick?

Let's take a look at how intermittent fasting improves your health.

***

Helps Losing Weight And Belly Fat

Most of the people who take up intermittent fasting do it with the main aim of losing weight. Intermittent fasting ensures that there is a restriction in your food intake. You will end up consuming fewer calories on this diet if you don't try to compensate for the fasting dates on the dates that you can eat.

It also helps in enhancing the function of hormones for facilitating better weight loss. Intermittent fasting not only helps in improving your metabolism, but it also helps in cutting down the calories you consume. Most of the weight that is shed is from the abdominal cavity.

***

Reduces Risk of Cancer

Studies in animals have shown that fasting starves cancer cells, making them vulnerable for destruction by your immune system. Fasting also protects healthy cells from chemotherapy toxicity.

A research group is now even working towards making make intermittent fasting an adjuvant therapy for cancer patients by trying to get the US Food and Drug Administration's (FDA) approval.

When Tim Ferriss interviewed Dominic d'Agostino, an associate professor at the South Florida Morsani College of Medicine, on the relationship between fasting and cancer, he said the following: *"If you don't have cancer and you do a therapeutic fast 1 to 3 times per year, you could purge any precancerous cells that may be living in your body."*

This is a good enough reason in and of its own to start intermittent fasting!

***

Positive Changes In Cell Functioning

When you don't consume food for a while, you do not just lose weight. There are many other positive things that also happen within your body.

For instance, the process of cellular repair and regeneration starts. There are changes in the hormonal levels in your body for making fat available for providing energy. While fasting, your insulin level drops. This facilitates fat burning. The level of growth hormones increases. And there is a positive change in the composition of several genes and molecules that support longevity and immunity against diseases.

***

Reduces Insulin Resistance

One of the most common forms of diabetes that can be tackled with intermittent fasting is Type 2 diabetes.

In this condition, the levels of blood sugar are high, resulting in resistance to insulin in the body. Unlike Type 1 diabetes (which is genetic), Type 2 diabetes is a reversible condition. Anything that would help in reducing the resistance towards insulin will help in reducing the levels of blood sugar in the body.

It has been shown that intermittent fasting helps in reducing insulin resistance in the body. For example, one study that was conducted on diabetic rats has shown that fasting helps in protecting them from kidney damage and the other complications that accompany Type 2 diabetes.

**

Reduces Stress and Inflammation

Oxidative stress can lead to chronic inflammation, which in turn will push you one step closer towards aging and other chronic diseases. Oxidative stress occurs when unstable molecules react with other useful molecules like protein or DNA and damage them in the process.

There are several studies that show that intermittent fasting can successfully improve the body's resistance towards oxidative stress.

It's Good For Your Heart

One of the terrible problems plaguing humanity is heart disease. Most of the health markers are related to an increase or decrease in the risk associated with heart diseases.

Intermittent fasting helps in improving various risk factors like blood pressure, good cholesterol, level of triglycerides, and even control the levels of blood sugar.

***

Slows Down Aging

When you start fasting, the cells in the body start the process of waste removal. This process involves breaking down the dysfunctional cells and proteins within it. The process of waste removal is referred to as autophagy, a Latin word that literally means 'self-eating'.

Autophagy is the natural cleansing process of your body. It facilitates the removal of waste that has been building up in cells. If this internal repair system is not performing at its peak, you get fat, age faster and are prone to developing chronic diseases.

If it functions well however, the bodily damage that is a by-product of the huge number of daily cellular reactions is healed naturally. You will look your age, and feel much healthier too.

The bottom line is that intermittent fasting not only helps you lose weight, but can also do wonders for your health!

Are you getting excited about giving it a try?

If you are, then you will need to pick a method. There are different ways of incorporating fasting in your daily routine. In the next chapter, we will discuss the most common ones.

3. Intermittent Fasting Methods: Which One Is Right For You?

"I'm kind of like a middle mix between a warrior diet and a Paleo diet, so I only eat once a day and it's at night - so kind of like interval fasting. But I eat until I'm full, I eat as much as I want, and I really don't eat anything that you couldn't find, you know, 10,000 years ago."

Ronda Rousey, former UFC Women's Bantamweight Champion. Also first American woman to earn an Olympic medal in judo (bronze)

__Key Takeaway__: Many methods of Intermittent Fasting have been developed over the years. The method that fits you best depends on your personal needs. You can go through this chapter to decide which method that is.

Intermittent fasting has become quite trendy in the recent past. It offers a wide range of benefits. Given its popularity, there are different variations of intermittent fasting that have been cropping up. All these methods can be effective. However, there will likely be only one that would best fit your needs and lifestyle.

Let's take a look at the most popular methods of intermittent fasting:

- 16:8 Method
- 5:2 Method
- Eat-Stop-Eat
- Alternate Day Fasting
- Warrior Diet
- Skipping Meals Spontaneously

***

16:8 Method (Leangains)

With this method, you would fast for a period of 16 hours every day. The eating window is restricted to about 8 hours. Within this window, you can manage to squeeze in two or three meals. This is also known as Leangains and it was made popular by Martin Berkhan, a fitness expert.

It could be something as simple as skipping breakfast or not munching on anything after dinner. For instance, you can stick to eating your last meal before 8pm. Then make sure that you don't eat anything till noon the following day. This provides you with a fasting window of about 16 hours.

If you are a woman, you would do better to fast for a shorter duration of time. Don't let your fasting period go beyond 14-15 hours.

If you are one of those that feel hungry in the morning and are used to having breakfast every day, the 16:8 method can be hard, initially. Over time, your body will adjust though. If you are already used to skipping breakfast, then this method would be easy. You are basically already doing the 16:8 method.

You can have water, coffee, and other beverages that don't have any calories in it while you are fasting. When you do eat, try to stay away from all forms of junk food, and eat healthy, wholesome foods instead. This method won't give the best results if you binge on foods that have a high caloric value. It would be easier to stick to intermittent fasting if you consume low-calorie meals.

***

5:2 Method

While following this diet, you would eat normally on five days of the week and restrict the calorie intake to 500-600 calories on the other two days of the week. This diet is referred to as the 'Fast Diet' and was made popular by Michael Mosley, a British doctor, and journalist.

On the two fasting days, it is recommended that women should have 500 calories and men can consume 600 calories. For example, on the fasting days, you can eat two meals consisting of 250-300 calories each.

This diet is suitable for all those who feel that they cannot fast for the whole day and who would like to eat a little something.

***

Eat-Stop-Eat

This form of intermittent fasting requires one to fast for 24 hours, once or twice every week. Brad Pilon, a fitness expert has popularized this diet a few years ago.

You will need to fast for 24 hours in this diet. In practice, this would mean that if you had your dinner at 7 pm on Monday, you don't get to eat again until 7 pm on Tuesday. You can also do this from breakfast on a given day till breakfast on the following day.
Just make sure you fast for 24 hours; you can select the timings according to your convenience. The choice is yours!

You cannot consume any solid food during the fast. However, water, coffee, and other beverages that don't have any calories in them can be safely consumed.

If you are following this method because you want to lose weight, then you will need to eat normally during your feeding window. You should eat the sort of food you are used to eating, had you not been fasting.

The only problem with this method is the length of the window: fasting for 24 hours might be difficult for some people. You don't have to necessarily start out with this method. You can gradually progress from the 16:8 fasting model. The first stretch of the diet wouldn't be hard; it is only towards the end that this diet gets a little difficult to follow. This is where discipline and motivation will come in handy.

***

Alternate Day Fasting

Like the name suggests, if you take this approach you would fast every other day. There are different variations of this diet. Some variations allow you to eat about 500 calories on every alternate day, and the others require you to observe a strict fast on the fasting day.

Most of the lab studies that have been conducted to find the benefits of intermittent fasting have used some variation of the alternate day fasting method. A strict fast might sound rather severe and extreme. Depending upon your comfort level, you can adapt this diet to suit your needs. It is advisable that beginners don't immediately jump to this method. With this method of fasting, be prepared to go to bed hungry a few times every week.

***

Warrior Diet

Ori Hofmekler, a well-renowned fitness expert, is responsible for popularizing this diet. On the Warrior Diet, you would consume small quantities of raw fruit and veggies during the day and a single hearty meal at night. Essentially, you will need to fast throughout the day, and then you get to feast at night.

The feeding window extends to only 4 hours. This intermittent fasting variation was one of the first to become popular. While following this method of fasting, the food choices that you make should be similar to those on a Paleo diet. In short: unprocessed foods that our cavemen ancestors would have consumed.

***

Skipping Meals Spontaneously

There is no structured plan for this form of intermittent fasting. You can reap all the benefits offered by an intermittent fast without having to plan any elaborate meals. This is quite an easy variation to follow. You will simply have to skip meals spontaneously from time to time. Skip meals whenever you aren't hungry or when you are preoccupied with some work.

It is definitely a myth that people will need to eat every couple of hours. Your body won't start losing muscle or even shift into starvation mode if you go without food for a couple of hours. Our bodies have been designed in such a manner that we can go without food for prolonged periods of time. Missing one or two meals from time to time will not do your body any harm. In fact, it will give your body a break and provide you with an opportunity to cleanse it.

So, if you aren't hungry, you can skip one meal. Then depending on your hunger quotient, you can have a hearty lunch or dinner accordingly. However, you will need to make sure that the other meals that you consume are healthy.

***

These are the most common methods of intermittent fasting. If you are new to fasting, I suggest you start easy: the 16:8 Diet would be my recommended choice for you. A potential downfall that many of us face, whether it is with fasting, starting a business or anything in life really, is that we – in our enthusiasm – tend to take on too much and then get burned. If that were to happen to you, you may never fast again and would miss out on the many advantages of intermittent fasting.

So take it one step at a time. Start with the entry level method. And move on to a more demanding method from there, if you want to.

Your heart and toned waistline will thank you.

4. Who Should Not Fast?

"Now there are more overweight people in America than average-weight people. So overweight people are now average. Which means you've met your New Year's resolution."

Jay Leno

Key Takeaway: *Fasting has many positive effects on your health. However, fasting can be risky for some. If you have an eating disorder, are pregnant or have any medical condition, always consult your physician first before starting any of the intermittent fasting methods.*

The positive effects of fasting on your health are truly spectacular. However, this doesn't mean that fasting is suitable for everyone.

It is good for healthy adults to fast from time to time. It helps in cleansing the system. There is no reason why a healthy adult shouldn't fast.

However, if you have an eating disorder, you should especially refrain from any type of fasting. And if you are pregnant or have a medical condition, please always first consult your physician before starting a fast.

***

Eating Disorders

If you have got any eating disorders like anorexia or bulimia, you shouldn't fast. I'm serious here. People who suffer from one of these eating disorders already tend to fast more than is healthy for them.

If you have an eating disorder, or your closest family has suggested you have, please do not practice intermittent fasting. You are probably already low on energy, and fasting will just worsen these conditions. If you have your mind set on doing one anyway, I highly recommend you visit a physician or nutritionist first.

***

Pregnant Women

The effect of fasting on an unborn fetus hasn't been documented. However, some argue that when a woman fasts while nursing, the milk produced isn't as nutritious as it is supposed to be. There might not be a difference in the amount of milk produced, however, the nutrient content in it is apparently less.

***

Type 2 Diabetes

Fasting has been used to reverse the effects of Type-2 diabetes since ages. There is even scientific research supporting these claims. However, if you do have Type 2 diabetes, I still suggest you first consult your physician before following any form of fasting. Better safe than sorry!

***

Other Medical Conditions

For many medical conditions, intermittent fasting is perfectly fine and can even be beneficial. However, there are some conditions that would prohibit you from starting intermittent fasting.

If you have any health issues related to your liver or kidney, you shouldn't fast. If you suffer from bouts of weakness, are malnourished, anemic, frail, or simply exhausted, you also shouldn't fast.

When in doubt, consult your physician. Especially if you are dependent on any medication, have a weak immune system, high blood pressure, or a weak circulation.

***

Before and After Surgery

For many types of surgery, it is recommended – sometimes even required – to fast for 12-24 hours prior. The purpose is to prevent stomach acid or food entering your lungs by travelling back up from your stomach to the esophagus during general anesthesia. This is called pulmonary aspiration.

You should not fast after you have undergone a major surgery, or if you are recovering from any major illness. Instead, eat a healthy diet with lots of vegetables, giving your body the nutrients it needs to recover and heal. Follow the instructions from your physician, and consult him in case of doubt.

***

Mental Fear of Fasting

If you have a fear towards fasting, then it is advisable that you don't fast. Fear doesn't put you in the right frame of mind for fasting. This can, in turn, make the experience unpleasant or even harrowing. Fear is a strong emotion and it can alter the physiological makeup of an individual. Therefore, it would be better if you have an open mindset towards fasting. If you don't, then you better not try it.

***

Children

Most of the children these days don't need to eat as frequently as they do. However, this does not mean they need to engage in extended periods of fasting. Although fasting once in a while for short periods of time will not do them any harm, a healthy child doesn't have to fast. The only exception to this rule may be children who are overweight or obese.

A child's body is still growing and developing, and it needs enough of the right nutrients to do so. If you are a parent who would like to let his child experiment with intermittent fasting, or if you are a child yourself and are reading this book, it would be better if you first consult a doctor. Especially if you intend the fast to last for prolonged periods of time.

***

Observe these safety precautions and you can be confident that intermittent fasting will result in the many health benefits we covered earlier.

Fasting has been around for thousands of years. Views and opinions on its health effects have shifted over time. Yet, there are some persistent myths about fasting out there. You may even think some of them are true, and consequently hesitate to start intermittent fasting.

In the next chapter, let's take a look at each of those myths, and debunk them one by one.

5. Common Fasting Myths Debunked

"When you don't have food in your life, just for a day, it makes you realize you're lucky to have it the next day. So the day after fasting, the music that comes out will be very joyous."

Chris Martin, singer of Coldplay

Key Takeaway: *Fasting is very popular and in the recent years, it's been co-opted by popular culture. Because of this, a lot of new information about fasting has come up but not all of it is true. This chapter will debunk some common fasting myths that can be harmful.*

There are many popular myths about intermittent fasting. In this chapter, we will look at the ten most common myths:

1. You will become fat if you skip breakfast
2. Eating frequently will boost your metabolism
3. Hunger reduces if you eat frequently
4. Small meals can help you lose weight
5. Your brain requires a constant supply of glucose
6. Your body will shift to starvation mode
7. Your body can only make use of a limited amount of consumed protein

8. You will lose muscle
9. It's bad for your health
10. When you are not fasting, you will overeat

Is there any truth to these myths, or are they false? By the end of this chapter, you can answer this question for yourself. The information below is not only helpful in deciding whether intermittent fasting is something you want to incorporate in your diet, but also if people refer to one of these myths when they question your fast.

***

Myth#1: You Will Become Fat If You Skip Breakfast

Breakfast is considered to be the most important meal. There is a heated debate that has been going on since forever regarding how special and important breakfast really is.

People tend to believe that skipping breakfast leads to:

• extreme hunger pangs
• an increase in appetite
• cravings for food, and
• ultimately weight gain

And there have been a few observational studies that appeared to have found an apparent link between skipping breakfast and weight gain.

However, a 2014 study put this issue to an end. This 16-week long randomized clinical trial was conducted to see if there was any causal connection between eating or skipping breakfast and weight gain or loss. The result? Contrary to popular belief, skipping breakfast had no negative effect on weight loss.

So, there is nothing special about breakfast. And you will not bloat up like a balloon if you skip this meal.

***

Myth#2: Eating Frequently Will Boost Your Metabolism

People tend to believe that consuming small meals frequently will help in improving your metabolism rate.

It is definitely true that your body makes use of some energy for digestion and assimilation of the nutrients present in food. This is referred to as the thermic effect of food, or TEF. It accounts for about:

- 20-30% of the calories for burning protein
- around 10% of carbs, and
- about 3% of fat

The TEF can account for 10% of the total caloric value of the food consumed.

In the end, the number of calories you consume matter and not the number of meals you consume. Consuming six meals comprising of 500 calories each would have the same effect as consuming three meals of 1000 calories each. The thermic effect would be about 10% on an average. This results in the burning of 300 calories in either of the cases.

***

Myth#3: Hunger Reduces If You Eat Frequently

Another popular myth is that eating frequently helps in keeping hunger and cravings at bay. However, this isn't necessarily true.

If you keep increasing the amount of food you consume, then your craving for the same will increase too. The jury is still out: a couple of studies show that increasing the frequency of meals will lead to a reduction in hunger, other studies recorded no change, and again some others suggest that there can be an increase in the hunger levels of an individual.

One study showed that consuming three meals that are rich in protein are better at reducing hunger than consuming six small meals that are rich in protein. Well, this varies from one individual to the next one. If you feel that frequent snacking will keep hunger at bay, then it is a good idea to snack frequently. However, like mentioned earlier, this just depends on one individual to the next. Do your own experiment.

***

Myth#4: Small Meals Can Help You Lose Weight

Frequent meals don't contribute towards boosting your metabolism. They don't help in reducing your hunger either. If eating frequent meals has no impact on the equation of energy balance, then it definitely will not help you lose weight. This is also proven by several studies that show that the frequency of meals has no effect on the process of losing weight.

However, if you have noticed that eating frequently makes it easier for you to cut down on calories and not gravitate towards junk food, then in such a case perhaps you should follow it. In fact, the idea of eating frequently sounds horribly inconvenient if you have got to stick to a diet.

***

Myth#5: Your Brain Requires A Constant Supply Of Glucose

Some people honestly believe that not eating carbs frequently will hinder the functioning of our brains. This is based on the popular misconception that the brain can function only on glucose fuel.

However, one important fact is often left out of this equation. The body can easily manufacture glucose through a process referred to as gluconeogenesis. The body stores glycogen in the liver, which can always be made use of for supplying the brain with the energy it requires. The body produces ketones during a low-carb diet or during extended periods of fasting. These are used when the energy requirement of the brain switches from glucose to ketones.

So, during a long fast, you need not worry about the brain not being able to support itself on glucose. The brain can make use of ketones through a process referred to as ketosis. In ketosis, glucose is produced from burning fats and proteins. If you suffer from hypoglycemia, then make sure you meet your required intake of carbs.

***

Myth#6: Your Body Will Shift To Starvation Mode

Another popular myth is that your body will go into the starvation mode when you start intermittent fasting. This, in turn, would shut down its metabolic functions and hinder it from burning fat.

Long-term starvation can indeed reduce the burning of calories in the body. This is referred to as starvation mode or thermogenesis. Depending upon the intake of calories, your body will decide how many calories it can afford to burn. Thermogenesis is inevitable when it comes to weight loss.

However, there is no valid evidence that suggests that thermogenesis is a common state of the body while on intermittent fasting. In fact, fasting for short periods of time will help in increasing the metabolic rate of the body. During a short-term fast, there is a spike in the levels of norepinephrine (also called: noradrenaline). This, in turn, helps in breaking down the fat and promotes metabolism.

***

Myth#7: Your Body Can Only Make Use Of A Limited Amount Of Consumed Protein

There are some claims that the body can only use about 30 grams of the protein that are consumed in a meal. Another popular claim is that you will need to eat every two or three hours if you want to enhance your muscle gain.

Neither of these claims are supported by science. The most important factor that matters to your body is the total amount of protein you have managed to consume and not the number of meals over which it is spread.

***

Myth#8: You Will Lose Muscle

It is believed that while fasting, our bodies start burning muscle to provide fuel. This is bound to happen when you start dieting.

However, there is no concrete evidence that proves that this happens at an increased rate while on intermittent fasting. In fact, there are certain studies that show that intermittent fasting is relatively better for the maintenance of muscle mass.

When compared to continuous calorie reduction, the reduction of muscle mass was less in intermittent fasting. In one study, the participants had to consume the same number of calories they would normally consume. However, now they had to do so in just one meal: dinner. At the end of the trial, the researchers observed that these people had lost body fat and there was a decent increase in their muscle mass.

This fasting technique is popular among bodybuilders too. It helps them maintain their body muscle without increasing the percentage of fat. And it is even used by Wim Hof, aka The Iceman. In his book 'Tools of Titans', Tim Ferriss describes Hof's diet as follows: *"I expected a mutant such as Wim to have dietary tricks. When I asked him about his typical dinners, his answer made me laugh: "I like pasta, and I like a couple of beers, too. Yeah!" How can he function on this food? Genetics might play a role, but he also rarely eats before 6 p.m. and tends to eat one single meal per day.*

To use the lingo of the cool kids: He has practiced intermittent fasting for decades now."

***

Myth#9: It's Bad For Your Health

Some people think that fasting could be harmful to their overall well-being. This is nothing but a myth. As we saw earlier, intermittent fasting has many health benefits.

For instance:

- It helps in changing the expression of certain genes that help in improving longevity and providing better protection against diseases.
- It also provides a boost to your metabolism and reduces oxidative stress in your body.
- It helps in tackling inflammation and reduces the different risk factors for various heart diseases and conditions.
- It also improves your brain's well-being. Intermittent fasting boosts the production of BDNF, which stands for brain-derived neurotrophic factor. This helps in providing protection against mental conditions like depression.

Some people may think that fasting is harmful, but the many proven health benefits show that they are wrong.

***

Myth#10: When You Are Not Fasting, You Will Overeat

Some claims have been made that intermittent fasting won't be of any help if you want to shed weight. Why? Because you would overeat during the feeding window.

This isn't fully incorrect. It is partially true that people tend to feel quite hungry after they break their fast. Some will feel the need to compensate for all the calories that they didn't consume throughout the day.

However, this compensation isn't a complete one. One study shows, for example, that people who have fasted for one whole day end up consuming 500 extra calories on the following day. Intermittent fasting helps in reducing your overall intake of food and also boosts your metabolism. It doesn't increase your weight and instead helps you shed a few kilos.

Once you get used to eating at particular intervals, you will learn to control your hunger and fasting will definitely help you in losing weight.

***

With these common myths on intermittent fasting debunked, let's get practical. Next up we will go over what you can consume during the fasting window.

6. What Can You Consume During the Fasting Window

"Internal purification is the first, crucial step toward achieving maximum health and vitality. By cleansing your body on a regular basis and eliminating toxins from your environment, your body can begin to heal itself, prevent disease, and become more strong and resilient than you ever thought possible! I firmly believe the definition of a doctor should be one who teaches, not one who prescribes."

Dr. Edward Group III

Key Takeaway*: During the fasting window, you are allowed to drink liquids that don't contain any calories. Water, tea and black coffee do not interfere with the fast. Avoid anything that can spike your insulin levels, such as milk and sugar in your coffee, chewing gum and diet drinks. Also stay away from alcohol.*

Intermittent fasting means abstaining from consuming any calories. Simply limiting food consumption to a certain time window already does wonderful things for your body.

You are allowed to drink non-caloric liquids, because these don't break the fast. Be careful though: you may consume something that you think is okay, but actually starts the digestive process and ends the fast.

***

Water/Tea

There are some people that advocate eating proteins, fruits and vegetables while on a fast but, technically speaking, you are not fasting if you are eating anything. Even having a cup of tea with honey in it could be classed as breaking the fast. However, just because you can't eat anything doesn't mean you should avoid drinking.

The most important thing to drink during a fast is water, at least eight glasses per day as a minimum. Not only does this keep you hydrated, it can also help you to feel more satiated. Other drinks that are also okay to drink because they don't contain any calories are:

- black tea
- green tea
- herbal teas
- carbonated water, and
- black coffee

***

Coffee

Speaking of coffee: try to keep your caffeine intake as low as you can, no more than two cups per day. Too much is not good for you on an empty stomach and won't make you feel any better about not eating.

Watch out for the extra calories in milk and sugar. It might seem like a tough call to drink your morning coffee black but you will get used to it, especially when you start to see the benefits of your intermittent fasting regime kicking in. Adding a bit of cream here, a spot of sugar there or even a bit of honey can have the effect of breaking the fast and sending your insulin levels back up. That means your body is not getting the full benefit of the fast. If you are doing a 24-hour fast, keep in mind that this is only for one or two days of the week so be strong about it and push on. You can do it if you really want to.

There is another good reason to watch your caffeine intake. Caffeine is a diuretic and, unless you are regularly topping up with water, all those extra trips to the bathroom will take their toll. That headache you have when you first start an intermittent fasting regime? This is NOT dehydration (unless you are not drinking sufficient water). Instead, it is probably a caffeine headache.

***

Avoid Insulin Spikes

Avoid anything that is going to cause your insulin levels to spike. You know by now that insulin regulates how much fat is stored in your body. Keeping it low while you do your fast ensures that your body is able to release the fat stores around your waist and hips, so that fat can be used and burned, instead of increased in size.

***

No Chewing Gum

Some people advocate eating sugar-free gum while on a fast. And while humans have been chewing leaves and gum tree sap for many thousands of years, you should avoid all forms of chewing gum on a fast.

The regular type contains both sugar and calories. Chewing gum is often sweetened with corn syrup, also known as glucose syrup. Every time you eat a piece of this gum, your blood sugar levels rise.

The sugar-free kind isn't much better because of the artificial sweeteners in it. Moreover, some people have an intolerance to phenylalanine, which is found in the artificial sweetener aspartame.

The key thing to remember: avoid chewing gum altogether.

***

No Diet Drinks

The same goes for diet drinks, whether it's a can of diet soda or a cup of diet iced tea. Steer clear of it all together while you are fasting. While a can of diet soda, or a stick of sugar-free gum for that matter, don't have many calories, once again it comes down to the negative effect the harmful chemicals will have on your health. Diet soda has also been shown to actually raise insulin levels, which is the opposite of what you want.

***

No Alcohol

Alcohol is also not allowed during the fasting window. Similar to diet drinks, alcoholic drinks contain calories that break the fast. A bottle of beer or a glass of wine actually contain over 100 calories. And definitely stay away from a piña colada, which contains almost 500 calories!

***

Although one of the biggest benefits of fasting is the weight loss, it is also a good time to give your body a rest from the chemicals that are in so many of the foods that we eat on a daily basis. When it comes time to do a fast day, treat your body to a diet of fresh clean water, black coffee, and unsweetened teas.

At the end of the day, it is pretty simple to work out what you can and can't consume on a fasting day. If you have to ask yourself whether you can or can't have it, the answer is to steer clear of it. It's only for a set period of time, and it will do you no end of good to give your body that break.

Next up, the fun really begins: ten steps to create your plan and kickstart your own intermittent fasting adventure!

7. How To Get Started – 10 Steps To Create Your Intermittent Fasting Plan

"MERCHANT: 'And of what use are they? For example, fasting, what good is that?'
SIDDHARTHA: 'It is of great value, sir. If a man has nothing to eat, fasting is the most intelligent thing he can do. If, for instance, Siddhartha had not learned to fast, he would have had to seek some kind of work today, either with you, or elsewhere, for hunger would have driven him. But, as it is, Siddhartha can wait calmly. He is not impatient, he is not in need, he can ward off hunger for a long time and laugh at it.'"

Herman Hesse, excerpt from Siddhartha

__Key Takeaway__: It can be quite difficult to start on the path of fasting and it's very common to be intimidated by it. It's important to understand that intermittent fasting is a way of life and before you get started you need to be prepared for it. You can do this by creating an extensive and detailed plan.

Getting started with intermittent fasting might definitely seem quite intimidating. This diet is really helpful when you want to gain control over your eating habits and also shed excess kilos. However, when it comes to getting started with the diet, the intimidation quotient stays the same. It doesn't go away.

Before you get started, you need to understand that intermittent fasting isn't just a diet.

It is a *lifestyle*.

You will need to accept that this is a way of life, if you want to keep going. A lot of our life tends to revolve around eating. The kind of intermittent fasting method you opt for will define the kind of lifestyle change you will need to make.

So, let's get started with creating a plan to kickstart your intermittent fast!

***

Step 1: Select The Method Of Fasting

In Chapter 2. Intermittent Fasting Methods: Which One Is Right For You? you learned the most popular methods of intermittent fasting. Which one is the most suitable for you depends on your personality, goals and lifestyle. Choose one that would fit best into your life.

Let's say you are a morning person, you enjoy working out early and will faint if you have to wait all day to get your first meal.

In such a case, your feeding window needs to be somewhere in between 10 am and 4 pm. You can probably opt for a fasting method where you will need to fast for 24 hours. In this manner, you don't have to worry about the pressure of having to fast on a daily basis. The method you should opt for would be eat-stop-eat. You can follow the warrior diet if you think you can get through a whole day with just one meal at night.

Take a moment to reflect on your lifestyle habits. This will give you pointers to the right intermittent fasting method for you.

***

Step 2: Do Plenty Of Research

You will need to do plenty of research to figure out the *right* diet for you. Go through the information provided in this book, check if your priorities and needs would fit in any of the methods mentioned. And only then select the method that you think would work best for you.

Your research would depend on your goals. Before you begin, determine exactly what your goals are. If you want to change your body composition by increasing muscle mass and decreasing body fat, give the 16:8 method a go. Conversely, if you are more interested in anti-aging and disease prevention, do a 24 or 36 hours fast once a week.

No matter what you do, do not fast for more than 72 hours.

Step 3: Get The Tools

There are plenty of tools and applications that will help make life easier for you when you are just starting out with intermittent fasting. There are paid and free apps that will help you in keeping track of your fast.

Intermittent fasting is a trial and error method. You will not know what will work for you unless you give it a go. These applications will help you in keeping track of your eating periods and provide you with the information that you need.

You can also maintain a journal for tracking your progress. It definitely helps if you have got substantial proof to believe that the diet works.

***

Step 4: Start The Transition

Unless you are an all-or-nothing sort of a person, starting with intermittent fasting can be quite difficult. If you aren't used to fasting, then going without food for prolonged periods of time won't be an easy task.

You will need to slowly condition your body so that the transition into the diet will be smooth. You can slowly start cutting out sugars from your diet. Start filling yourself up on protein. Or drink a bulletproof coffee (with butter and MCT oil) in the morning. Fast for short periods of time; you can gradually increase your fasting time.

***

Step 5: Find The Necessary Support

Are you familiar with the proverb 'shared joy is a double joy; shared sorrow is half a sorrow'?

It would be helpful if you could start your intermittent fasting with someone else. It could be your partner, friend, or even a family member. Each can use the other as a coach and a support system. You can fast together and exercise together. Whenever you feel like giving up, there would be someone else to keep you motivated and make sure that you are on the right track. It is simpler to shop for groceries and plan your meals when you have company.

***

Step 6: Tone Down Your Workouts

Often times, potency requires minimalism. Much like the strength of coffee or any alcoholic drink dissipates as you dilute it with water, the efficacy of your workouts during intermittent fasting may follow suit if you train too much. But what does overtraining look like in this context?

The obvious examples are exercising at a very high intensity and for longer periods of time. When you exert too much effort (intensity) than what your body can currently handle under a fasting state, you run the risk of burning out, getting sick or being injured. Even at the right intensity, regularly working significantly longer than what your body can safely handle creates a similar risk as excess intensity. Can you imagine if you do both at the same time?

What does the right intensity look like? Generally speaking, you would feel very uncomfortable – lightheaded, very tired and weak or prolonged muscle soreness – during or after working out if you over train. A relatively objective way of determining if you're exercising at moderate intensity, which is ideal, is through the talk test. If you can still carry a normal conversation while working out albeit with some difficulty, that is moderate. If you are able to carry a conversation in the same manner as you would over coffee with a friend, or if you can barely say a word while catching your breath, then you are under (low intensity) or over (high intensity) training, respectively.

A good way to focus your training is to prioritize compound exercises, i.e., those that involve the most number of major muscle groups to execute the movements. Examples of these would be burpees, which recruit most of your major muscles groups.

Another way of prioritizing your exercise is to go for those that utilize the biggest muscle groups, particularly legs and back. Why? The bigger the muscles, the more calories are required to contract them. That's why doing 1,000 crunches aren't enough to get you ripped but running daily for at least

30 minutes, which involves the biggest muscle group that's the legs, can help you do so.

***

Step 7: Follow Delayed Gratification

Delayed gratification is a brilliant technique to make use of. It works extremely well with intermittent fasting.

If your co-workers at your workplace have got some yummy sweet treats to work and you are extremely hungry, your mind will tell you to give in. When the hunger pang strikes you, even a bowl of frosted cereal with cold milk seems quite appetizing. All that you will need to tell yourself is that you can definitely eat all that, but not at the given point of time. You can even write down the list of foods that you had denied yourself.

This will not only help you in staying focused, but it will also stop your mind from obsessing over the foods that you cannot eat.

***

Step 8: Protein Should Be A Priority

Always make sure that you have your proteins and complex carbs before anything else.

There might be something sweet or oily on your eating list. However, eating those before anything else can prove to be quite problematic. If you consume such items first, you will end up overeating. Not only are these foods rich in calories, the amount of nutrients is also minimal. All that you will end up with is a tummy ache.

Planning your meals ahead will be very helpful. Just make sure they have sufficient protein and complex carbohydrates in them. It is likely that you will start craving for these things by the time your feeding window approaches.

Make sure that you fill yourself up with grilled chicken, lentils, or any other form of proteins, and some healthy vegetables. You can include a little bit of carbs in the form of sweet potatoes, potatoes, a serving of rice, or something starchy.

After you have consumed all this, there will be little or no space left for any form of junk food. Your hunger will force you to fill yourself up with the good stuff and you won't binge on unhealthy junk.

***

Step 9: Take A "Before" Photograph

Before you get started with intermittent fasting, the one thing that you need to do would be to take a photograph of yourself. This would be the "before" photograph.

This will help you in getting started with the diet, and keep on keeping on when the going gets tough. You can gauge your progress by comparing yourself to the image. This will definitely make you want to keep going. Your weight might not reduce immediately, but you can slowly see the fat giving way to lean muscle.

***

Step 10: One More Thing To Keep In Mind

If you are just getting started with intermittent fasting or you want to give this diet a go, you will need to keep in mind one important thing.

The initial phase of this diet is the hardest to get through. The initial two weeks are the toughest and after that, it does get easier. These first weeks are the toughest because your body is just getting used to the fasting schedule. You will slowly start to gain control over your cravings, hunger pangs, and your appetite too. It can take anywhere from a few days to a few weeks for your body to get acclimatized to the diet.

So, give yourself some time and let your body get used to the diet.

***

With these ten steps, you have everything you need to lay a solid foundation to successfully implementing intermittent fasting in your daily routine.

But what would your weeks look like?

8. Intermittent Fasting Plan Templates

"My first meal is at 2 p.m. And then I eat from 2 to 10. Over the last five years, I've been doing intermittent fasting. Now, within the times I don't eat, the fasting period, which is a 16-hour fasting, I drink amino acids drinks. I'll have coffee, maybe tea. Now, the problem with intermittent fasting is that you never want to have a bad meal. Because you're, like, "I waited all day, 16 hours for this?". Over the last five years it's really kept me in great, great shape. I can feel the difference. I literally can put pictures of myself now versus pictures of myself at 22 years old, and I look and feel much better right now."

Terry Crews, former NFL star, and host of Netflix's 'Ultimate Beastmaster'

Key Takeaway: If you're ready to start with Intermittent Fasting then you have to create a template. A template for fasting is nothing but a schedule which gives you directions in terms of when you have to fast and when not to.

Now that you know what intermittent fasting is all about, the next step is to write down what you want to achieve, create a fasting template and follow it.

***

Write Down Your Goals

If you have followed the ten steps to creating your own intermittent fasting plan, you now know why you want to start intermittent fasting. Take a pen and paper and write your goals down. Studies show that writing down your goals significantly increases the chance of accomplishing those goals.

If possible, be specific. If a goal is measurable, you will be able to tell if you have accomplished it. For example, the goal 'I want to feel good' is not measurable. Your mood can change per day, regardless of your diet. However, the goal 'I will lose 5 lbs in 5 weeks' is a measurable goal: you can weigh yourself now, as well as 5 weeks from now, and see if you have hit your target.

Once you have written down your goals, next you will need to create a plan for the intermittent fasting method you plan to follow.

***

16:8 Method (Leangains)

If you want to follow the Leangains method of intermittent fasting, you will have to get used to fasting on a daily basis. The plan for this method is quite simple.

Make sure that most of your fasting time falls within your sleeping period. You will have to fast for 16 hours per day. If you sleep 8 hours a night, that already covers half of that. The simplest form would be to fast for four hours before going to sleep and four hours after waking up.

Let's say you go to bed at midnight. Then, you would stop eating at 8 pm. The next day, you can break your fast around noon, and have until 8pm before your next 16 hour fast begins.

Here is what it would look like:

Timings	Sunday	Monday	Tuesday	Wednesday	Thursday	Friday	Saturday
Midnight	Sleeping and fasting	Sleeping and fasting	Sleeping and fasting	Sleeping and fasting	Sleeping and fasting	Sleeping and fasting	Sleeping and fasting
8 am	Fasting	Fasting	Fasting	Fasting	Fasting	Fasting	Fasting
Noon	Feeding window	Feeding window	Feeding window	Feeding window	Feeding window	Feeding window	Feeding window
8 pm	Fasting	Fasting	Fasting	Fasting	Fasting	Fasting	Fasting
Midnight	Sleeping and fasting	Sleeping and fasting	Sleeping and fasting	Sleeping and fasting	Sleeping and fasting	Sleeping and fasting	Sleeping and fasting

This schedule will be repeated on a daily basis. The only feeding time available for you will be that eight-hour window.

***

68

5:2 Method / Eat – Stop – Eat

With the 5:2 method, you will need to reduce your caloric intake to 500-600 calories for two fasting days in a week. The starting time does not really matter: you can choose to start your fast after dinner or after breakfast. As long as it lasts for 24 hours.

The following template is for a fast that starts in the night:

Sunday	Monday	Tuesday	Wednesday	Thursday	Friday	Saturday
Eat normally	Start fasting after dinner. Around 8pm in the night	Fast till 8pm in the night	Eat normally	Start fasting after dinner. Around 8pm in the night	Fast till 8pm in the night	Eat normally

***

The Warrior Diet Method

This is a very easy template to make. You will need to fix a feeding time for yourself at night. This is the only time when you will get to eat a proper meal, although you are allowed to munch on a few healthy snacks during the fasting window, like raw fruits and vegetables.

On the Warrior Diet, your week would look something like this:

Timings	Sunday	Monday	Tuesday	Wednesday	Thursday	Friday	Saturday
Midnight	Sleeping and fasting	Sleeping and fasting	Sleeping and fasting	Sleeping and fasting	Sleeping and fasting	Sleeping and fasting	Sleeping and fasting
8 am	Fasting	Fasting	Fasting	Fasting	Fasting	Fasting	Fasting
8 pm	Feeding window	Feeding window	Feeding window	Feeding window	Feeding window	Feeding window	Feeding window
Midnight	Sleeping and fasting	Sleeping and fasting	Sleeping and fasting	Sleeping and fasting	Sleeping and fasting	Sleeping and fasting	Sleeping and fasting

***

You now know everything you need to pick your preferred intermittent fasting method and get started!

Like with any lifestyle change, there will be challenges ahead after the initial excitement wears off. How do you stay motivated and on track to ensure you experience the long-term benefits of intermittent fasting? That's what we will discuss next.

9. How To Stay On Track and Motivated

"Our bodies are our gardens – our wills are our gardeners."

William Shakespeare

Key Takeaway*: Fasting is difficult and many people give up on it due to a lack of motivation to continue. Staying on track requires you to stay positive and apply some simple techniques that will ensure that you don't get disheartened easily.*

The main reason why most of the diets fail is because of lack of motivation. Most people tend to start a diet with a lot of motivation, and then as time passes by, this motivation starts to fade away. Intermittent fasting is no different.

Motivation starts to fade away when you don't get the results you expected or you don't get them soon. The results you hoped to get will take a while and this causes your motivation level to take a nosedive.

Here are a few tips and tricks that will help you to stay focused and motivated, so you can accomplish the goals you set when you started intermittent fasting.

***

Don't Expect Results Overnight

The one thing that you should remember is that you won't get any instant results. No diet provides you with instantaneous results and it is not good for you in the long run.

Did you gain those extra 10 pounds over night? No, you didn't.

So, what makes you think that you will be able to shed them overnight? It takes a while.

This doesn't mean that the diet isn't working. It simply means that it will take a while to tone your body. You will not be able to achieve the perfect body that you hoped for in a week's time. A diet, when combined with exercising, provides you the results you hoped for, after a while. It takes more than a while. So, be patient and don't give up.

At times, it really does get difficult to keep going. There might be some temptation lurking around the corner or you simply feel disheartened. Regardless of what the reason is, here are three things that you can do to make sure you stay motivated.

If you are not seeing the results you were hoping for, it may be time to review your diet and lifestyle. What some people forget is that a fast is not the only thing that will help. Many other factors affect the way you lose weight, and the amount. You have to look at intermittent fasting along with other healthy habits, like exercise and sleep, which will ensure that you lose weight consistently.

***

Use Positive Affirmations

You now know not to expect miracles in just a short time. Well, this may seem easy in theory but chances are you will start feeling terrible when you find no changes after a week or two.

This is when you will need to motivate yourself and tell yourself that you are doing a great job. You have to keep forging ahead and will need to give yourself the strength to stick to the fasting method.

Write down a few positive affirmations related to your fasting goals and repeat them out loud every day. Here are some examples of positive affirmation you could use:

- It does not cost me any effort to practice intermittent fasting, it is so simple!
- I can easily resist any temptation to stop my fasting method
- I am so proud of myself that I am working on improving my health
- I love the feeling of successfully completing yet another fast!

If you repeat these affirmations on a daily basis, your brain *will* believe you. These are mantras to trick your brain!

***

Measure Your Progress Using a Mirror Instead of a Scale

Start off by making use of the mirror and not the scale to measure your progress.

As you start your diet, you should stand in front of the mirror right after taking a shower. A full-length mirror would be ideal. Notice the areas from where you want to lose weight and the places where you want well-sculpted muscles. Capture a mental picture of yourself. This would be your "before the diet" body. You can watch it change as you start following the diet.

Why don't you take a picture of yourself and keep this in view to motivate yourself every time you feel like giving up? It would serve as a reminder to stay on track. It will also work as a positive encouragement for you. You can gauge your progress by comparing yourself to the image. This will definitely make you want to keep going. Your weight might not reduce immediately, but you can slowly see the fat giving way to lean muscle.

***

Partner Up

One of the steps to creating an intermittent fasting plan is finding the necessary support. This is also crucial for staying motivated.

If you have to do it all on your own, without any support, staying on track will require a lot more willpower and persistence. And numerous studies have shown that willpower is a depletable resource. If this is your defense to challenges, well, good luck to you!

But if you have the support of someone else who is in the same boat, that will make all the difference. Most of the times, when you feel like giving up, your partner will be there to pick you up and push you back in the right direction. And when he or she is struggling, you will be there to return the favor.

Also, you can use positive affirmations to motivate each other, like: 'Practicing intermittent fasting with you feels effortless, I am so happy that we are doing this together!'

***

Eat Healthy, Delicious Foods

Make sure that you include a variety of healthy, yummy foods in your diet. Just because you eat healthy and abstain from food for certain periods of time does not mean you need to suffer!

No one likes to eat the same thing every single day. It gets boring and repetitive. There are millions of healthy recipes available online which you can make use of. Modify them to suit your needs and requirements. If you become bored with the food, you will lose the motivation to continue. Address this before it even becomes a possible issue and intermittent fasting will be a breeze!

You have the power to get the body you always wanted. It takes motivation, focus, and some patience. Discipline yourself to stick to the diet and keep on pushing yourself. All your hard work will definitely pay off.

***

Stay Calm and Keep it Cool

You will have to get rid of your thoughts about the number of hours you can fast. Stop asking yourself if you should only fast for nine instead of ten hours! Stop worrying about how consuming a single French fry during your fasting period is going to affect it.

If this happens, please relax. You have an extremely smart body, which will adapt itself to any changes you may make to your lifestyle.

If you are looking at consuming lunch or breakfast one day and want to skip it the next, go ahead. If you are aiming to become an athlete or aiming towards becoming strong and muscular, you will need to be very rigid with respect to your diet. Otherwise, you should just chill!

***

Do Not Worry About People Staring at You

When you first start intermittent fasting, you may at some point find yourself in a situation where people give you that weird look. For example, when you are out for lunch with your colleagues and your plate remains empty.

Now, what do you tell them? You will probably have to take a lot of time to explain yourself. Use what you have learned about the common fasting myths we debunked earlier. But if they do not understand what you are saying, then embrace the weirdness!

This is the time where you can revert to your goals and regain focus. Why are you practicing intermittent fasting? What you wrote down on that piece of paper is what matters, not the approval of colleagues. If people around you support you, that is great! But if they don't, do not let them sidetrack you. Once you have accomplished your goals, you will be the one laughing.

***

Keep Yourself Busy

If you have just started your intermittent fasting routine, you will probably have trouble trying to curb your thoughts about hunger. You may sit around and begin to wonder about how hungry you are. And you will probably crave for some form of food.

Let me give you a plan that you could use during the first few days of your fast.

Right before the first few hours of your fast, you should consume a huge meal! Let's call it a monster meal. You will stop worrying about when you are going to eat next. You could try sleeping a decent amount of time since you cannot worry about hunger when you are dreaming! Try to keep yourself busy during the day to avoid worrying about your hunger. Last, but never the least, keep telling yourself that you do not need to think about hunger since you are a strong person!

***

Always Listen To Your Body

Each person has respond differently to intermittent fasting. You will never be able to gauge how your body will react to the fasting by comparing yourself with people around you. You will need to see how your body reacts and then make the changes required.

Are you concerned about losing too much muscle mass? If so, start keeping track of your strength by undertaking strength training routines to assess the intensity of your strength. You could buy fat calipers that would help you track how well the fat has started to burn away in your body. Always keep a track of your caloric intake! You will be able to see how your body has started to change with respect to the quantity of food you eat.

Final Words

There you have it: all the information that you need about intermittent fasting.

Thank you again for reading this book, *'Intermittent Fasting: Burn Fat, Lose Weight And Build Muscle With Ease While Still Eating Your Favorite Foods!'*

I hope you feel comfortable – and excited! – to incorporate everything you have learned into your own diet.

By reading this book you have learned:

- What intermittent fasting is
- The many health benefits of intermittent fasting
- The different intermittent fasting methods you can choose from
- If fasting is right for you
- How to debunk 10 popular fasting myths
- What you can consume during the fasting window
- 10 steps to get started and create your own intermittent fasting plan
- Intermittent fasting plan templates, and
- How to stay motivated and on track

Despite the popular belief that not eating for prolonged period of time is not healthy, the truth is that it actually creates amazing health benefits. And once you have adapted to the fast, you won't even feel hungry.

The trick for getting it right with intermittent fasting is to eat properly and make sure that you are eating the right foods during your feeding window. During your fasting period, make sure that you are consuming plenty of fluids and are keeping your body well hydrated.

Intermittent fasting has got so many benefits; I really encourage you to give it an honest chance. If one intermittent fasting diet doesn't give you the results you long for, try another method. For example, if you are fasting for 24 hours twice a week, consider trying the 16:8 method. It would be ideal if make sure that your fasting period coincides with your naptime. If you work during nights, make sure that your fasting time falls within the timeframe of your sleep.

Now the next step is to apply what you have learned. This can be a challenging process at times. We all have our moments of weakness. Take it one step at a time. And don't beat yourself up if you temporarily fall off track. Nobody is perfect! Success is simply a matter of getting up one more time than you fall.

Resources

Books

- Brad Pilon – Eat. Stop. Eat
- Ori Hofmekler – The Warrior Diet
- Herbert M. Shelton – Fasting Can Save Your Life

***

Websites

- Leangains.com
- Bradpilon.com
- Eatstopeat.com
- Jamesclear.com/the-beginners-guide-to-intermittent-fasting
- Reddit.com/r/leangains
- Precisionnutrition.com/intermittent-fasting
- Thefastdiet.co.uk
- Theiflife.com

***

Documentaries

- Live Long Die Young
- Eat Fast and Live Longer

Podcasts

- Greatist Podcast - Brad Pilon on Intermittent Fasting, Mindful Eating, and Why Chocolate is Great
- Primal Blueprint Podcast #3 – Intermittent Fasting with Mark Sisson
- Bulletproof Podcast #174 - Brad Pilon: Eat Stop Eat & the Fundamentals of Intermittent Fasting

BONUS CHAPTER: The Health Benefits of Juicing

Below, you will find a free bonus chapter from my book **'Juicing For Beginners***: Feel Great Again With These 50 Weight Loss Juice Recipes!'*

It is my way of saying thanks for:

- *Reading this book, and*
- *Taking your health seriously. You rock!*

Let's get started, shall we?

***

"He that eats till he is sick must fast till he is well."

English Proverb

Key Takeaway: Fruit and vegetables contain a lot of healthy nutrients. Through juicing you increase your fruit and vegetable nutrient intake. Juicing results in many health benefits. It slows down aging, makes you look better, helps you lose weight, increases your energy level, and boosts your immune system.

Introduction

An average adult should consume:

- two to three servings of fruit, and
- three to five servings of vegetables a day

At least, that is what many nutritionists, doctors, and government agencies recommend.

According to the Centers for Disease Control and Prevention (CDC):

*"Compared to people who eat only small amounts of fruit and vegetables, those who eat more generous amounts — as part of a healthy diet — are likely to have **reduced risk of chronic diseases**. These diseases include stroke, Type 2 diabetes, some types of cancer and perhaps heart disease."*

How many servings do you eat per day?

You are probably not surprised when I tell you that most people don't come anywhere close to these recommendations.

But here is the **health hack**: juicing provides an effective and simple way to meet your dietary requirements for fresh fruit and vegetables! Just adding one glass of fresh juice to your daily diet can make all the difference!

Sounds good, right?

But wait, there is more. Juicing is not only good for disease prevention. In this chapter, we are going to take a quick look at all the many benefits of juicing.

***

Juicing Slows Down Aging

As you grow older, your body starts to lose strength and energy. Grey hairs appear, or you may even start to lose hair.

An important cause of aging are free radicals, which damage cells. As a result, these cells become more vulnerable to premature aging and disease. This process cannot be prevented entirely, aging is inherent to life. But what you can do is feed the cells nutrients of the highest quality. This will strengthen them, and enable them to perform at an optimal level. Remember the Ferrari analogy?

Fruit and vegetables are full of those superpower nutrients. And if you juice them, you are not only able to consume more of the good stuff per day, your body will also absorb the nutrients more easily. How does this work?

As years go by, your digestive system starts taking hits from all the toxins that enter your body as a result of all the bad foods you eat. Think KFC, muffins and soft drinks. This impairs your body's ability to properly digest the food you eat and absorb all its nutrients. Even if it's healthy food! But by juicing the food, you have already done most of the digesting before you even take your first sip. Compare it to baby food: because of its soft texture, it is easier for the baby to digest. By juicing fruit and vegetables, you allow the nutrients to pass directly into your bloodstream. It's like injecting natural doping!

***

Juicing Makes You Look Better

As you start to juice on a daily basis, you will notice that your skin starts to improve. Your skin is one of the biggest bodily organs, and consists of three layers:

- **Epidermis**: this is the outer layer, which provides a waterproof barrier to external toxins and chemicals, as well as the sun's rays. It also gives your skin its color.

- **Dermis**: this deeper layer provides the epidermis with new cells, as dead cells are flaked off its surface. It produces oil to keep your skin soft, it grows hair and produces sweat.

- **Hypodermis**: this is the deepest layer. Among other things, it stores fat and controls your body temperature.

The nutrients in fruit and vegetables, as well as the water in them, improve the quality of the cells in your skin. During the first days of a juice fast, you may see some acne or pimples pop up, but that is a good sign: your skin is going through a process of purification, expelling toxins. But shortly after, you will start noticing your skin transforming. It will start glowing more, while wrinkles and facial lines are lessening.

And the effects of juicing on your body doesn't stop there. Your hair and nails, which are directly connected to your skin, will also become stronger and begin to shine more.

Who doesn't want to look good? With juicing, you will not only feel healthier, but you'll also be welcomed by a prettier face in the mirror in the morning. Plus, you will be able to save a lot of money on all kinds of beauty products, yay!

***

Juicing Helps You Lose Weight

In the introduction of this book, I told you how Joe Cross lost 82 pounds in 60 days of juice fasting. And I have personally lost 13 pounds a number of years ago when I did a 10-day juice fast. And the best thing is: most of it stayed off, after I returned to a normal diet!

Losing weight is simply a matter of burning more calories than you take in. Your body will then start using the fat already stored in your body as fuel, and burn it. Fruit and vegetables contain carbohydrates and plant proteins, but no fat. Just a reminder: fat isn't categorically bad for you. Your body needs a small amount of healthy fats, especially Omega-3 fats are good for you. These can be found in foods like salmon, walnuts and soybeans. However, by building your diet around fruit and vegetables, you will keep your fat intake low.

Just by replacing eating potato chips or Oreo cookies with drinking a green smoothie, the pounds will start flying off!

***

Juicing Increases Your Energy Level

To perform at an optimal level, your body needs to be in a prime state. And the way to get there is to give it what it needs: high-quality nutrients. Juicing is one of the best ways of doing so. Juiced fruit and vegetables contain the building blocks of healthy cells, such as vitamins, potassium and antioxidants. And because you juice them, they are injected in the bloodstream almost immediately after you drink it. You will be able to think more clearly, feel more vital, your memory improves, and you will feel better about yourself.

There is even a mental effect. I like to jog in the park. When I get tired, I try to pump myself up again and keep going. One way of doing that is by simply raising my arms in the air, like athletes do when they win a race. But another thing I have experimented with is visualizing a healthy juice. And the effect is really interesting: when I visualize French fries, or other unhealthy foods, my energy level drops even further. But when I visualize a healthy green smoothie, it energizes me. Try it out for yourself!

***

Juicing Boosts Your Immune System

Your body is an impressive superorganism. It is exposed to a variety of toxins, bacteria and viruses every day, yet you don't get sick most of the time. Why is that? Because of your powerful immune system. The immune system is the body's first line of defense, and it keeps most unwelcome visitors out.

The stronger your immune system, the better it can perform. And the less sick you will be. Fruit and vegetables are jam-packed with phytochemicals. These are chemicals that plants produce to protect themselves. But they can also prevent, or mitigate the effects of, diseases in humans. So, by juicing fruit and vegetables, you are strengthening your immune system, and laying the foundation for a healthy life.

Additionally, juicing is also great to detox the body, especially if you do a juice fast. Juicing allows your body to clear waste from the digestive system and your liver, as well as rid your body of all kinds of toxins.

***

Now you know the most important health benefits of juicing. But what do you need to make a juice? You will need a powerful juicer that is able to distract all the nutrients from the fruit and vegetables, without crushing them. That's why I recommend you use a proper juicer, and not a blender.

Next up, you will learn the difference between a juicer and a blender.

***

This is the end of this bonus chapter.

Want to continue reading?

Then get your copy of "Juicing for Beginners" at your favorite bookstore!

Did You Like This Book?

f you enjoyed this book, I would like to ask you for a favor. Would you be kind enough to share your thoughts and post a review of this book? Just a few sentences would already be really helpful.

Your voice is important for this book to reach as many people as possible.

The more reviews this book gets, the more people will be able to find it and improve their health through intermittent fasting.

***

IF YOU DID NOT LIKE THIS BOOK, THEN PLEASE TELL ME! You can email me at **feedback@semsoli.com**, to share with me what you did not like.

Perhaps I can change it.

A book does not have to be stagnant, in today's world. With feedback from readers like yourself, I can improve the book. So you can impact the quality of this book, and I welcome your feedback. Help make this book better for everyone!

Thank you again for reading this book and good luck with applying everything you have learned!

I'm rooting for you...

About The Author

Hi, my name is Gerard Hamilton. Thank you once again for reading this book. I am a nutritionist and fitness enthusiast, and I am extremely passionate about health. I am the author of bestselling books, such as 'Juicing For Beginners' and 'Intermittent Fasting'.

Having been overweight myself when I was younger, I know the struggles that many of my readers face every day.

The million-dollar question is: How can you lose weight *and* enjoy life at the same time?

Well, that is what I am here to teach you!

It is my purpose in life to help you become the best possible version of yourself. This is what makes me come out of bed every morning.

So join me on this journey and let me help you take back control of your health, lose weight and have some fun while we are doing it.

Happy reading!

By the Same Author

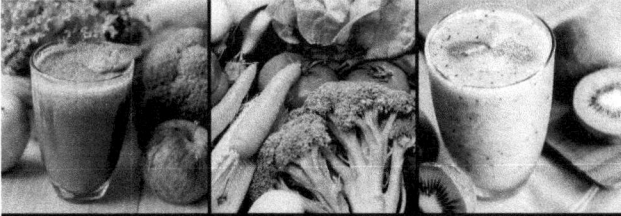

JUICING FOR BEGINNERS

FEEL GREAT AGAIN WITH THESE 50 WEIGHT LOSS RECIPES

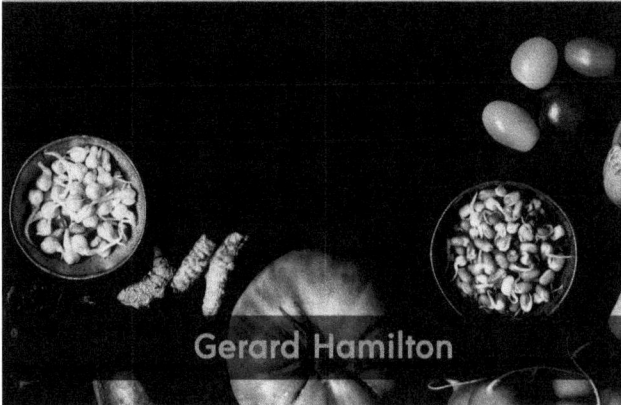

Gerard Hamilton

Notes

www.ingramcontent.com/pod-product-compliance
Lightning Source LLC
Chambersburg PA
CBHW071241020426
42333CB00015B/1574